YOUR KNOWLEDGE HAS VALUE

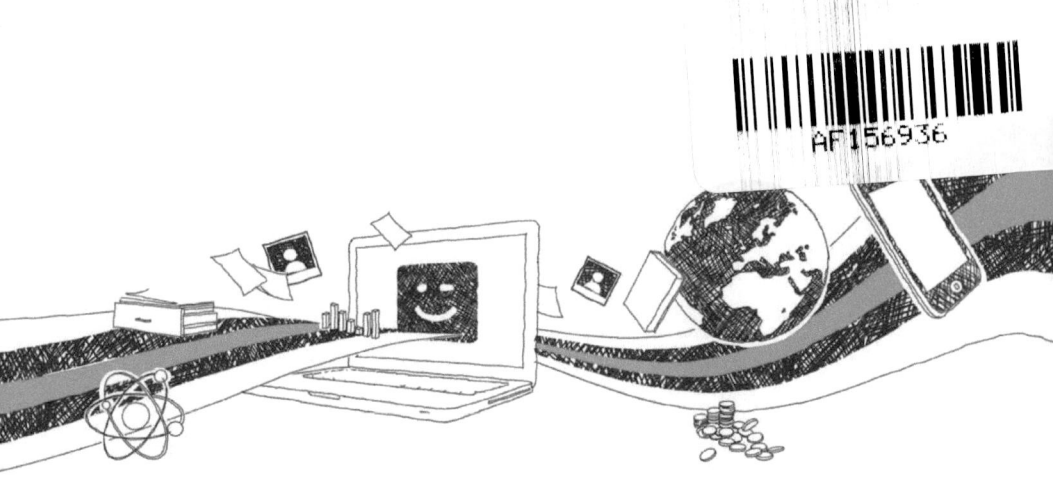

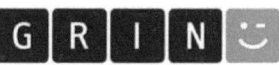

Bibliographic information published by the German National Library:

The German National Library lists this publication in the National Bibliography;
detailed bibliographic data are available on the Internet at http://dnb.dnb.de .

Imprint:

Copyright © 2015 GRIN Verlag, Open Publishing GmbH
Print and binding: Books on Demand GmbH, Norderstedt Germany
ISBN: 9783668307032

This book at GRIN:

http://www.grin.com/en/e-book/336695/improving-the-work-life-balance-of-regis-
tered-nurses

Maren Düchting

Improving the Work-Life Balance of Registered Nurses

GRIN Publishing

GRIN - Your knowledge has value

Since its foundation in 1998, GRIN has specialized in publishing academic texts by students, college teachers and other academics as e-book and printed book. The website www.grin.com is an ideal platform for presenting term papers, final papers, scientific essays, dissertations and specialist books.

Visit us on the internet:

http://www.grin.com/

http://www.facebook.com/grincom

http://www.twitter.com/grin_com

Executive Summary

The Mater Private Hospital is the biggest hospital of Mater Health Services. Its main strengths are the long tradition and good reputation due to a high healthcare quality. The focus on high quality is also positioned in its vision to become the leader of compassionate and exceptional healthcare. Currently, reaching the vision is at risk. Due to a poor work-life balance the job satisfaction as well as motivation of nurses decreased. In addition, high stress levels lead to a poor nursing outcome and impair the healthcare quality. Furthermore, an increasing turnover rate causes lowered organisational cost efficiency and high recruitment costs.

An internal and external analysis of the labour market, the MPH, and the role of nurses, showed the great importance of a good WLB, a high commitment and a high retention rate. Since one of MPH's main goals is to continually improve its employment offer in order to increase the retention rate, it is recommendable that it implements an intervention that increases the WLB, job satisfaction and retention rate.

Two possible interventions have been examined: (1) Flexible Working Hours and (2) Mentoring Programme. The recommended intervention for the MPH is implementing a Mentoring Programme. It shows the same advantages in its outcome as the flexible working hours (higher job satisfaction, better WLB, higher commitment). However, it has more advantages than flexible working hours: it also improves older nurses' retention, improves the team environment, and improves the knowledge and education of younger nurses. Therefore, it contributes to achieve the MPH's vision by increasing the healthcare quality.

A generated action plan, including key actions, success criteria, timescales, resources, responsibilities, monitoring and evaluation against success criteria shows a detailed implementation strategy. After the implementation it is recommendable according to the CHRM framework to continually assess and improve the mentoring programme.

Table of Contents

1 Introduction... 1

   1.1 Background and Purpose 1

   1.2 Methodology 1

   1.3 Limitations.. 2

2 Situational Analysis 2

   2.1 Labour Market... 2

   2.1 Mater Private Hospital... 3

   2.2 The Role of RNS... 3

3 Interventions.. 4

   3.1 Intervention 1 – Flexible Working Hours 4

      3.1.1 Rationale 4

      3.1.2 Advantages and Disadvantages.. 5

   3.2 Intervention 2 – Mentoring Programme... 5

      3.2.1 Rationale 6

      3.2.2 Advantages and Disadvantages.. 6

   3.3 Recommended Intervention.. 7

4 Action Plan 8

5 Conclusion... 10

References... 11

Appendices.. 14

1 Introduction

The following report recommends the Mater Private Hospital (MPH) intensive care unit (ICU) to implement a mentoring programme. It will not only improve registered nurses' (RNS) work-life balance (WLB) and increase the retention rate but also improve the RNS' education and therefore increase the likelihood of achieving the MPH vision.

1.1 Background and Purpose

The MPH belongs besides several hospitals and health centres to the Mater Health Services. It is the biggest of Mater Health Services' hospitals with over 328 beds, and 96,623 patient days in 2014 (Mater Health Services 2014). In order to take care of the high number of patients, to meet the patients' expectations and maintain the good reputation, the MPH has a great need of a large number of highly committed and qualified nurses.

The current issues of bad working conditions and poor WLB are severe weaknesses of the MPH. Increased stress and lowered motivation among the RNS can negatively affect the patient care and therefore the MPH's reputation (Appendix 1). Furthermore, increased absenteeism- and turnover rates cause high replacement and recruitment costs. To maintain the good reputation, reduce costs and therefore stay competitive the MPH has a great need for an intervention that improves the nurses' WLB and consequently increases motivation, commitment and the retention rate.

1.2 Methodology

The methodology is based on the CHRM decision-making framework (Härtel & Fujimoto 2010). To perform the six steps, two different approaches have been applied. Firstly, an environmental analysis generated a SWOT and GAP analysis (Step 1) (Appendix 1; Appendix 2). Therefore, the MPH's needs, and possible risks could be figured out (Step 2). Secondly, a literature review resulted in and assessed two possible interventions (Step 3). In consequence one intervention was chosen and an implementation action plan, including success and against success criteria, was developed (Step 4-6).

1.3 Limitations

The report contains two main limitations. Firstly, the access to MPH's data was limited. Therefore, an overall and in-depth data analysis was not possible. Secondly, the report does not focus on possible costs of the interventions.

2 Situational Analysis

In order to get an in-depth understanding of the main issue of a high turnover rate due to bad working conditions, a detailed external (labour market) as well as an internal (Mater Private Hospital) analysis is required. Additionally the role of RNS is examined to understand nurses' needs and their importance for the MPH.

2.1 Labour Market

Australia faces an overall shortage of nurses (Dawson et al. 2014; Appendix 1). Taking into consideration that the demand for nurses increased between 2001 and 2011 with an upward trend the shortage signifies a severe issue to the health care sector (ABS 2013). Therefore, hospitals are going to have increasing issues when recruiting highly qualified nurses (Appendix 1). Implementing a mentoring programme or flexible working hours can result in both attracting applicants and retaining employed nurses. Thereby, the risk of having an insufficient number of nurses is lowered, and the MPH can avoid high costs interrelated to recruiting.

Another issue is the ageing workforce (Jackson & Daly 2004; Buchan & Aiken, 2008; Appendix 1). In 2011 one third of Australian nurses was 50 years or older. Regarding the data from 2001 the ageing process within the workforce also shows an upward trend (ABS 2013). Due to the increasing age the risks of health issues among the workforce increase. In order to avoid early withdrawals from the workforce or early retirements due to health issues the MPH is demanded to implement health-promoting measures and prevent stress or fatigue that could negatively affect the state of health. Flexible working hours or mentoring programmes can avoid health affecting working conditions. Thereby, high recruitment costs can be avoided and experienced nurses and their knowledge retain in the MPH.

2.1 Mater Private Hospital

Two of MPH's main strengths are a long tradition, and a good reputation (Appendix 1). MPH's vision is to become the leader of compassionate and exceptional healthcare (Mater Health Service 2014). The current issues regarding RNS can have severe impacts on the vision. High turnover rates across nurses affect the nursing care outcomes and therefore the quality of healthcare (Hayes et al. 2012; Appendix 2). Furthermore, it causes high financial losses. A nurse's withdrawal results in costs estimated between $42,000 and $64,000, including separation, recruitment, and replacement (Barton, Gowdy & Hawthorne 2005; Hayes et al. 2012).

Due to high stress levels, a poor WLB, and high turnover rates the MPH has to face many negative effects like lowered job satisfaction, decreased nursing quality, decreased efficiency, increased error rates, unsatisfied patients, and therefore a damaged reputation (Hayes et al. 2012). To achieve the vision, increase the organisational cost efficiency, and fulfill the self-defined goal to continually improve the employment offer the MPH has to implement an initiative that improves the WLB and the retention rate (Appendix 2).

2.2 The Role of RNS

Although the number of nursing students has increased since 2001, many young nurses decide to transfer to another organisation or change their profession due to bad or overstraining working conditions (Barton et al. 2005; ABS 2013; Dawson et al. 2014).

Australian nurses are confronted with high physical, mental, and emotional demands since they are responsible for the patient care and patients' wellbeing (Birks et al. 2013). Although nurses have a great responsibility their wages are relatively low (ABS 2013; Deans 2014).

Work-life strains are often caused by shift work since it affects nurses' psychological, physiological health, and their social lifes (Grzywacz et al. 2006; Perrucci et al. 2007; Skinner et al. 2011). Especially the high number of female nurses (90% in 2011) with children struggle (ABS 2013). It can be seen in a higher absenteeism rate during school holidays.

Many RNS are confronted with stressful situations, e.g. aggressive patients (Deans 2014). Moreover, they experience many traumatic incidences, e.g. deadly diseases, dolour or despair which can lead to psychological stress (Honkavuo & Lindström, 2014). Another stress factor is the strong social commitment. Many nurses put others' needs and interests above their own. Consequently, their WLB is affected and their stress level rises (Mullen 2015). Therefore, it is the MPH's responsibility to provide initiatives that create a WLB.

3 Interventions

To improve the WLB and therefore to increase the retention rate, two interventions are possible: (1) Flexible Working Hours and (2) Mentoring Programme.

3.1 Intervention 1 – Flexible Working Hours

There are different types of flexible working hours. The model that should be applied in the MPH includes temporal flexibility and a re-arrangement maintaining the total amount of working hours (Costa & Sartori 2005).

3.1.1 Rationale

One of the main reasons why nurses' work-life balance is negatively affected is the working time (Skinner et al. 2011). Shift and night work was found to cause health problems, and issues in social lifes (Costa & Sartori 2005). Firstly, it results in sleep disturbances, and fatigue which does not only have impacts on nurses' wellbeing but also on the organisation since it increases the risk of errors (Costa & Sartori 2005). Secondly, due to night, weekend and holiday shifts the social life of nurses can be highly impaired as the interaction to family and friends is affected (Grzywacz et al. 2006; Perrucci et al. 2007). Studies have shown that not the duration but the arrangement of working hours causes issues, and high stress levels (Barnett 2006).

Implementing an individual-oriented flexibility regarding working hours can lead to lowered stress levels as the nurses are able to adjust their working time to their specific needs (Costa & Sartori 2005). An individual- or employee-oriented flexibility means that the nurses are allowed to codetermine their working hours by planning breaks, holidays, and starting and end times (Beckers et al. 2012). Two possible systems that could be implemented in the MPH are self-scheduling and flextime (Beckers et al. 2012).

3.1.2 Advantages and Disadvantages

Flexible working hours have many advantages for both the organisation and the employee. Firstly, the nurses get a higher self-determination which enables them to adapt their work to their private life schedules (Beckers et al. 2012). Secondly, more flexibility results in a better well-being and a greater job satisfaction (Costa & Sartori 2005). Thirdly, stress can be decreased since nurses can match their recovery with their effort (Beckers et al. 2012). Overall, flexible working hours lead to an improved WLB which results in higher commitment, motivation, and consequently in an increased retention rate.

Some disadvantages have to be mentioned. Firstly, implementing flextime or self-scheduling applies to every employee and is therefore a change process. Change processes can result in uncertainty, resistance and even more stress (Harris et al. 2010). Secondly, particularly in the beginning it can take the nurses a lot of time to plan their schedules individually. In order to improve the WLB they should be allowed to do it during their working time. This could lead to a financial loss for the MPH. Thirdly, there is a risk that the nurses do not come to an agreement what can cause conflicts.

3.2 Intervention 2 – Mentoring Programme

Usually mentoring is known as spontaneous, informal partnerships. A mentoring programme for the MPH is an employee development tool that creates an organised and formal partnership (Lach et al. 2013).

3.2.1 Rationale

A mentor can function as role model for his mentee (Sharma & Freeman 2014). He can act as a friend, teacher, facilitator, coach, and consultant (Smith, McAllister & Snype Crawford 2001; Pulce 2005). Therefore, the mentee can confide in his mentor and discuss stressful situations as well as traumatic experiences. By giving both career- and social-related support mentoring focuses on personal and organisational aspects (Young & Perrewé 2000). Therefore, the mentor can support his mentee with advices regarding the WLB as well as in handling difficult emotional situations in the workplace. In addition, he can teach his mentee and thereby improving the nursing outcome and the healthcare quality.

Supportive colleagues and working in a good team environment can make nurses having a greater job satisfaction and can cause in a will to stay in the hospital (Cameron & Brownie 2010). Therefore, the support of mentors can result in a higher retention rate. For the MPH's mentoring programme it is recommendable that older, experienced nurses act as mentors and have younger, stressed nurses as mentees.

3.2.2 Advantages and Disadvantages

A mentoring programme can have many advantages for the organisation, the mentor, and the mentee (Petersen et al. 2012). Firstly, mentoring results for the mentee in both higher subjective career outcomes (e.g. higher commitment, lowered stress level) and higher objective outcomes (e.g. enhanced clinical competency, higher compensation) (Smith et al. 2001; Allen et al. 2004; Bulut, Hisar & Demir 2010). Secondly, the mentor will experience social recognition from managers and colleagues (Young & Perrewé 2000). Thirdly, the MPH will profit by the overall increased job satisfaction among mentees and mentors, a higher commitment as well as an increased retention rate. Furthermore, a better education results in a higher healthcare quality. Therefore, the MPH will be more likely to fulfil its vision.

Possible disadvantages can arise from a poor planning and implementation. Due to the complexity of the relationship mentor and mentee have to match regarding their personalities (Young & Perrewé 2000). In case the mentor and

6

mentee do not get along with each other the programme is likely to fail. Moreover, the mentors have to be aware of a power misuse that could cause anxiety instead of lowered stress levels (Smith et al. 2001).

3.3 Recommended Intervention

The MPH should implement a mentoring programme due to several reasons. On the one hand, it has the same outcome as flexible working times: higher job satisfaction, increased motivation, and higher retention rates. On the other hand, it has additional benefits.

Firstly, it is voluntary. Due to a restricted data analysis, it could not be figured out if every nurse has a need for a WLB initiative. Secondly, it does not only focus on young nurses with children but also on older nurses who get an additional benefit by experiencing recognition. Flexible working time could pose the risk of disadvantaging childless nurses. They could be forced by their colleagues to take night, weekend and holiday shifts. Mentoring creates a supportive and good team environment instead of provoking conflicts. Thirdly, difficult situations cannot be eliminated on nurses' workplaces. They always have to deal with difficult patients or traumatic experiences. Mentoring can help to build up resilience and cope with those situations. Fourthly, experienced nurses can teach inexperienced nurses and improve their knowledge which causes a higher healthcare quality. Thereby, the MPH is more likely to achieve its vision.

4 Action Plan

Action	Success Criteria	Time-scales	Resources	Responsibility	Monitoring	Evaluation against Success Factors
Nurses Needs Assessment and Intervention Presentation to Board of Directors and Executives	- ≥ 85% response rate - ≥ 50% high stress levels - ≥ 50% poor WLB - ≥ 50% interest in mentoring programme - Directors' approval	Week 1-3	- Data (turnover rate, absenteeism) - Survey Program - Statistics Program - Presentation Program (e.g. PowerPoint) - Meeting room (with projector) - Handouts for directors	- HR Unit - *Administration*	- Everyday report about response rate - Survey Email reminder to employees - Survey results to HR director min. 3 days before presentation date	- Evaluation of response rate - Questionnaire Evaluation - Voting after presentation
Task Force Formation Program and Finance Planning	- 5-10 employees in Task Force *Mentoring* - Finance Plan meets budget restrictions - Approval of CFO and CEO - Coherent Mentoring Programme	Week 4-6	- Budget plan - Finance software - Employees in Finance Department - Research possibilities - Software to create Mentoring Programme - Mentoring expert (e.g. consultant)	- HR Director - Task Force *Mentoring* - HR Unit *Employee Development* - Finance Unit	- The Task Force *Mentoring* is responsible and has to give a weekly report to the HR Director - HR Director reports weekly on Executive board	- Comparison Finance Plan with total budget - Presentation to CEO and CFO - Programme assessment by Mentoring expert
Mentor Recruitment and Training Mentee Selection and Questionnaire	- 1 : 1 number of mentors : number of mentees - Mentors improve cognitive and social skills - ≥ 95% training attendance - ≥ 95% applications of interested nurses of first survey	Week 7-10	- Personnel files - Announcement - Competence profile for mentors - Trainer - Rooms for training - Teaching resources (checklists, handouts, booklets)	- Task Force *Mentoring* - HR Unit *Recruitment* - HR Unit *Talent Management* - Staff Unit *Training*	- HR *Recruitment, Talent Management,* and *Training* Unit report on Task Force - Task Force *Mentoring* processes data and reports on HR Director - HR Director reports weekly on Executive board	- Comparison applications mentors and mentees - Pre- and post-test (cognitive and social factors) - Attendance lists - Comparison mentee applications and interested nurses of first action

8

Phase	Targets	Timeline	Resources	Responsible	Process	Evaluation
Mentor and Mentee Matching, Testing Phase	- Personality and needs of mentees match with mentors - ≤ 5% complaints after week 16 - 100% response rate - 100% interview attendance	Week 11-16	- Rooms for interviews - Survey Software - Statistic Software - Presentation Software to process data - Licence for personality questionnaire - Interviewer - Complaint management system	- Task Force *Mentoring* - HR Unit *Administration*	- HR *Administration* reports on Task Force - Task Force *Mentoring* processes data and reports on HR Director - HR Director reports weekly on Executive Board	- Personality questionnaire (e.g. Big Five) - Expectations and needs assessment (Questionnaire) - Interviews with mentees and mentors - Analysis and documentation of complaints
Mentoring Observation and Assessment	- Turnover rate reduces - Absenteeism rate reduces - Job satisfaction and motivation increase - High patient satisfaction - ≥ 90% Mentoring focuses on nurses' needs and expectations - ≤ 3% complaints	Week 17-24	- Rooms for interviews - Personnel data - Survey software - Statistic software - Complaint management system - Licence for job satisfaction questionnaire	- Task Force *Mentoring* - HR Unit *Employee Development* - Quality Management - HR Unit *Administration*	- HR *Employee Development*, and *Administration* report on Task Force - Task Force *Mentoring* processes data and reports on HR Director and Quality Management - HR Director reports on Executive Board	- Patient survey - Observing data and statistics - Interviews with mentors and mentees - GAP analysis of needs and expectations questionnaire and current status - Questionnaire job satisfaction
Assessment and Improvement	- Approx. 12% turnover rate - Approx. 15% absenteeism - No absenteeism increase during school holidays - Lower stress level - Better WLB - Good reputation - Higher cost efficiency	Week 24 onwards	- Licences for Questionnaires - Personnel data and statistics (pre and post mentoring) - Financial data and statistics (pre and post implementation) - Data formatting software	- HR Director - Task Force *Mentoring* - HR Unit *Employee Development* - Finance Unit - Executive and Director Boars - HR Unit *Administration*	- HR *Employee Development*, *Administration*, and Finance Unit report on Task Force - Task Force *Mentoring* processes data and reports on HR Director and Quality Management - HR Director reports on Executive Board	- Comparison of data before and after the implementation - Questionnaire evaluation about WLB, stress and job satisfaction and comparison with data before the implementation - Media coverage - Financial Analysis

5 Conclusion

Regarding external and internal factors, a poor WLB and a high turnover rate are serious threats for the MPH. By implementing a mentoring programme the hospital can increase the job satisfaction, motivation, WLB and retention rate. In addition, a mentoring programme can improve the healthcare quality and is therefore an initiative that can result in the fulfillment of the MPH's vision. An important part of the implementation is the regular evaluation against success factors. Since the CHRM framework is a dynamic tool the mentoring programme should be continuously tested and improved.

References

Allen, TD, Eby, LT, Poteet, ML, Lentz, E & Lima, L 2004, 'Career Benefits Associated With Mentoring for Protégés: A Meta-Analysis', *Journal of Applied Psychology*, vol. 89, iss. 1, pp. 127-136.

Australian Bureau of Statistics (ABS) 2013, *Australian Social Trends, April 2013, Doctors and Nurses*, viewed 25 October 2015, <http://www.abs.gov.au/AUSSTATS/abs@.nsf/Lookup/4102.0Main+Features 20April+2013>.

Barnett, RC 2006, 'Relationship of the Number and Distribution of Work Hours to Health and Quality-of-Life (QOL) Outcomes', in Perrewé, PL & Ganster, DC (ed.), *Employee Health, Coping and Methodologies*, Research in Occupational Stress and Well-being vol. 5, Emerald Group Publishing Limited, pp. 99-138.

Barton, DS, Gowdy, M & Hawthorne, BW 2005, 'Mentorship Programs for Novice Nurses', *Nurse Leader*, vol. 3, iss. 4, pp. 41-44.

Beckers, DGJ, Kompier, MAJ, Kecklund, G & Härmä, M 2012, 'Worktime control: theoretical conceptualization, current empirical knowledge, and research agenda', *Scandinavian Journal of Work, Environment & Health*, vol. 38, no. 4, pp. 291-297.

Birks, M, Cant, R, James, A, Chung, C & Davis, J 2013, 'The use of physical assessment skills by registered nurses in Australia: Issues for nursing education', *Collegian (Royale College of Nursing, Australia)*, vol. 20, iss. 1, pp. 27-33.

Buchan, J & Aiken, L 2008, 'Solving nursing shortages: a common priority', *Journal of Clinical Nursing*, vol. 17, iss. 24, pp. 3262-3268.

Bulut, H, Hisar, F & Demir, SG 2010, 'Evaluation of mentorship programme in nursing education: A pilot study in Turkey', *Nurse Education Today*, vol. 30, iss. 8, pp. 756-762.

Cameron, F & Brownie, S 2010, 'Enhancing resilience in registered aged care nurses', *Australasian Journal on Ageing*, vol. 29, iss. 2, pp. 66-71.

Careers at Mater Health Service 2015, viewed 24 October 2015, <https://careers.mater.org.au>.

Costa, G & Sartori, S 2005, 'Flexible work hours, ageing and well-being', *International Congress Series*, vol. 1280, June 2005, pp. 23-28.

Dawson, AJ, Stasa, H, Roche, MA, Homer, CSE & Duffield, C 2014, 'Nursing churn and turnover in Australian hospitals: nurses perceptions and suggestions for supportive strategies', *BMC Nursing*, vol. 13, iss. 11, pp. 1-10.

Deans, C 2004, 'Who cares for nurses? The lived experience of workplace aggression', *Collegian*, vol. 11, iss. 2, pp. 32-36.

Gilley, A, Waddel, K, Hall, A, Jackson, SA & Gilley, JW 2015, 'Manager Behavior, Generation, and Influence on Work-Life Balance: An Empirical Investigation', *The Journal of Applied Management and Entrepreneurship*, vol. 20, iss. 1, pp. 3-23.

Grzywacz, JG, Frone, MR, Brewer, CS & Kovner, CT 2006, 'Quantifying Work-Family Conflict Among Registered Nurses', *Research in Nursing and Health*, vol. 29, iss. 5, pp. 414-426.

Harris, R, Bennett, J, Davey, B & Ross, F 2010, 'Flexible working and the contribution of nurses in mid-life to the workforce: A qualitative study', *International Journal of Nursing Studies*, vol. 47, iss. 4, pp. 418-426.

Härtel, CEJ & Fujimoto, Y 2010, *The CHRM model and decision-making framework*, Human Resource Management, Pearson, Frenchs Forest, pp. 14-34.

Hayes, LJ, O'Brien-Pallas, L, Duffield, C, Shamian, J, Buchan, J, Hughes, F, Spence Laschinger, HK & North, N 2012, 'Nurse turnover: A literature review – An update', *International Journal of Nursing Studies*, vol. 49, iss. 7, pp. 887-905.

Honkavuo, L & Lindström, UÅ 2014, 'Nurse leaders' responsibilities in supporting nurses experiencing difficult situations in clinical nursing', *Journal of Nursing Management*, vol. 22, iss. 1, pp. 117-126.

Jackson, D & Daly, J 2004, 'Current Challenges and Issues Facing Nursing in Australia', *Nursing Science Quarterly*, vol. 17, iss. 4, pp. 352-355.

Lach, HW, Hertz, JE, Pomeroy, SH, Resnick, B & Buckwalter, KC 2013, 'The Challenges and Benefits of Distance Mentoring', *Journal of Professional Nursing*, vol. 29, iss. 1, pp. 39-48.

Mater Health Services 2014, *Health. Education. Research. 2014 Annual Review*, Brisbane, viewed 24 October 2015, <http://www.mater.org.au/Files/Documents/Corporate/Mater-Health-Services-Annual-Review-2014.pdf>.

Mater Hospital 2015, viewed 24 October 2015, <http://www.mater.org.au/>.

Mullen, K 2015, 'Barriers to Work-Life Balance for Hospital Nurses', *Workplace Health & Safety,* vol. 63, no. 3, pp. 96-99.

Murray, P & Syed, J 2005, 'Critical issues in managing age diversity in Australia', *Asia Pacific Journal of Human Resources*, vol. 43, iss. 2, pp. 210-224.

Perrucci, R, MacDermid, S, King, E, Tang, C, Brimeyer, T, Ramados, K, Kiser, SJ & Swanberg, J 2007, 'The Significance of Shift Work: Current Status and Future Directions', *Journal of Family and Economic Issues*, vol. 28, iss. 4, pp. 600-617.

Petersen, R, Eggert, A, Grümmer, R, Schara, U & Sauerwein, W 2012, 'The mentoring of women for medical career development', *International Journal of Mentoring and Coaching in Education*, vol. 1, iss. 2, pp. 155-168.

Pulce, R 2005, 'What Is a Mentor?', *Nurse Leader*, vol. 3, iss. 4, pp. 9-10.

Roberts, RK & Grubb, PL 2013, 'The Consequences of Nursing Stress and Need for Integrated Solutions', *Rehabilitation Nursing*, vol. 39, iss. 2, pp. 62-69.

Sharma, GV & Freeman, AM 2014, 'Mentoring Why it Matters Even After Training', *Journal of the American College of Cardiology*, vol. 64, iss. 18, pp. 1964-1965.

Skinner, N, van Dijk, P, Elton, J & Auer, J 2011, 'An in-depth study of Australian nurses' and midwives' work-life interaction', *Asia Pacific Journal of Human Resources*, vol. 49, no. 2, pp. 213-232.

Smith, LS, McAllister, LE & Snype Crawford, C 2001, 'Mentoring Benefits and Issues for Public Health Nurses', *Public Health Nursing*, vol. 18, iss. 2, pp. 101-107.

Young, AM & Perrewé, PL 2000, 'The exchange relationship between mentors and protégés: the development of a framework', *Human Resource Management Review*, vol. 10, iss. 2, pp. 177-209.

Appendices

Appendix 1 – SWOT / TOWS Analysis   p. 15

Appendix 2 – GAP Analysis   p. 16

Appendix 1 – SWOT / TOWS Analysis

	Strengths 1. long tradition 2. good reputation 3. high quality patient care 4. multiple clinical areas 5. leader in health, education, research 6. good location 7. good transport connection 8. lived values 9. emphasis on education and development 10. dynamic & multi-disciplinary teams 11. professional and personal support 12. employee benefits (e.g. gym, cafes, parking, child care centre)	**Weaknesses** 1. low employee retention rate 2. increasing absenteeism 3. high stress level 4. low motivation and engagement 5. reduced organisational cost efficiency 6. poor work-life balance 7. heavy responsibility 8. health risk 9. shift-work 10. low wages
Opportunities 1. Support by the Australian government (Private Health Insurance Rebate) 2. Technological advancements which simplify the work 3. Ageing population causes older people and more patients: increasing profit 4. Increasing awareness regarding to health 5. Good ratings, award winning	**SO Strategies** Maxi-Maxi Strategies Strategies that use strengths to maximise opportunities e.g. train the employees to use the technological advancements	**WO Strategies** Mini-Maxi Strategies Strategies that minimize weaknesses by taking advantage of opportunities e.g. using the increasing profits caused by the ageing population to invest in a work/life balance strategy
Threats 1. High number of competitors (e.g. Brisbane Private Hospital, St. Vincent's Private Hospital) 2. Costs for education & trainings 3. Costs for highly qualified employees 4. Generation X and Y ask for more work-life balance 5. Ageing workforce 6. Labour market shortage 7. Decreasing organisational loyalty 8. Decreasing well-trained employees	**ST Strategies** Maxi-Mini Strategies Strategies that use strengths to minimize threats e.g. promote the long tradition and good reputation to weaken the competition	**WT Strategies** Mini-Mini Strategies Strategies that minimize weaknesses and avoid threats. e.g. implement a work-life balance strategy to attract Generation X and Y

Careers at Mater Health Service 2015: Mater Hospital 2015: Gillev et al. 2015: Murrav & Sved 2005

Appendix 2 – GAP Analysis

Critical HR Issues at „Mater Private Hospital, Brisbane, intensive care unit (ICU)":

Unsatisfactory work-life balance among registered nurses

Current Critical Issues / Status Quo	Gap and Remedies to address critical issues	Desired Status & Outcomes	Evidence of Success
• High employee fluctuation • Increased absenteeism rate (especially during school holidays) • High work load and stress level • Lack of motivation and work engagement • Costly recruitment procedures to get highly trained nursing staff • Insufficient work-life balance initiatives • Dissatisfied patients	• Difference between current and ideal state because of a critical work-life balance among the registered nurses • Introducing work-life balance friendly programs, e. g. flexible working arrangements, job-sharing, part-time contracts, employee assistance programs, mentoring programs etc.	• Low employee fluctuation due to improved staff retention • Decreased and constant absenteeism rate • Moderate work load and stress level by means of appropriate resources • Motivated and engaged employees • Reduced recruitment and organizational costs • Implementation of work-life balance interventions • Satisfied patients	• 90 % retention rate • Turnover rate approx. 12% • Less than 15 % absenteeism • Monitoring stress level by a workplace stress questionnaire • Overall 95 % staff satisfaction by survey • Reduction of recruitment and organisational costs by 25 % • Overall 95 % patient satisfaction measured by follow up survey

YOUR KNOWLEDGE HAS VALUE

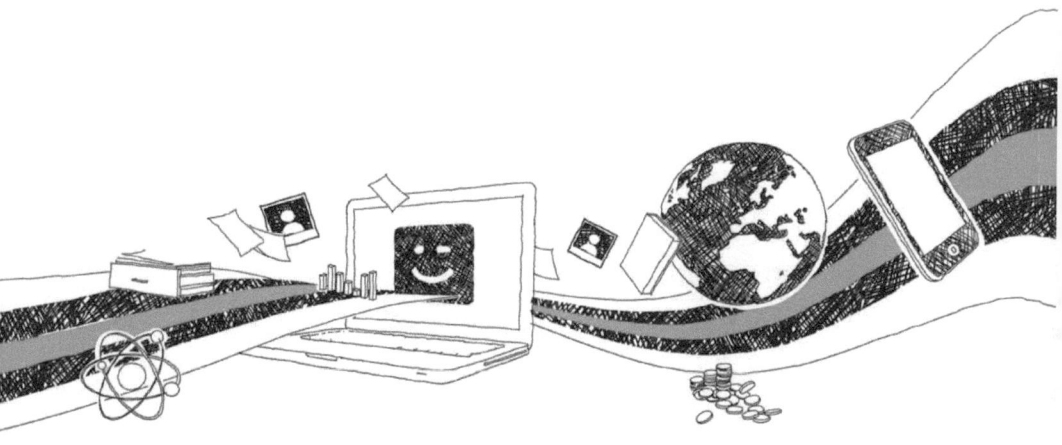

- We will publish your bachelor's and
  master's thesis, essays and papers

- Your own eBook and book -
  sold worldwide in all relevant shops

- Earn money with each sale

Upload your text at www.GRIN.com
and publish for free

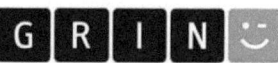